OLD DISEASES ARE COMING BACK

COURTESY OF

ANTI-VACCINATORS

BY

Amy Miller

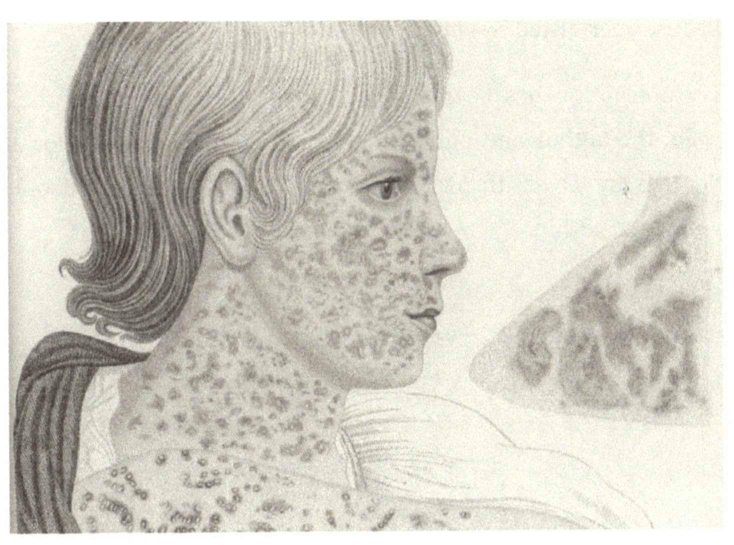

Table of Contents

Introduction

The term "vaccine" is derived from "Vacca," a Latin word meaning "horse." This unique name derives from the following historical event. Edward Jenner, a physician, observed a peculiar trend that the milkmaids who developed cowpox were later immune to smallpox.

In 1796, to confirm his hypothesis, he took some contaminated cowpox matter and revealed another healthy boy through a cut in his leg.

The kid got cowpox. Upon recovering from this simulated infection, he then injected him to smallpox, but the boy remained healthy. He invented the first cow-named vaccine.

Each parent in the world wants to do the best for their kids; their primary focus is to keep their kids safe from harm. But unfortunately, many parents don't know that the best way to protect their children is to vaccinate them.

Most parents are concerned with the concept of vaccinating their child or not, so here's a brief explanation of when vaccines are developed and what function they serve.

There is no adequate evidence as to who invented vaccination, it might be Persians, Chinese or Indians.

Yet Edward Jenner developed the first vaccine for smallpox. Since then, medical science has continued to evolve and medical researchers have created vaccines for many diseases including rabies, tetanus, polio, cholera, tuberculosis, typhoid, etc.

The reason for creating vaccines was to protect people from life-threatening diseases. Vaccination is inserted into a person's body's bloodstream; vaccination is sometimes offered at an early age, while in some instances it should be repeated after a few month intervals.

In this ebook, I will look at the pros and cons of vaccination, discussion on both sides of the issues.

Chapter 1

In many families, childhood and teenage immunizations are unclear. This is a simple guide to help parents understand vaccines.

What's vaccination or immunization?

The immune system detects pathogens (germs) as foreign substances when entering the skin. Doctors call these foreign substances antigens, and when they enter the body, the immune system develops antibodies to fight antigens. Immunizations (also called vaccines) include damaged or dead antigens.

The antigens in our bodies cannot generate the signs or symptoms of the antigen that cause infection, but they stimulate the immune system to create antibodies.

These antibodies help protect and defend your child against possible exposure to the disease. Immunizations not only help keep your child safe and healthy they also benefit all kids around the country and the world by stamping out major childhood diseases.

Is vaccination safe?

Vaccines are usually very healthy, Lawant to Brock says. Protection by immunizations greatly outweighs the very low risk of severe problems. Vaccines have made most dark and serious childhood diseases rare and sometimes kill (meaning extinct) the pathogen so that it is no longer around.

Does vaccination cause autism?

Vaccines are extensively studied and the CDC tells us they cannot cause autism. Despite a lot of speculation, researchers have not found a connection between autism and childhood immunization.

Yes, the initial study that sparked the controversy years ago was removed. Because signs of autism that occur at about the same time as children receive such vaccinations, it is because this is the developmental period doctors discover. It's just a coincidence, and you shouldn't worry about getting sick from these immunizations.

Will vaccines have side-effects ?

Some immunizations at the injection site can cause mild temporary side effects including fever, irritability, or soreness. Researcher Lawant to Brock advises that your child may grow a lump under the skin of the shot. The healthcare professional will speak to you about possible side effects with certain vaccines.

When is my baby immunized?

The generic guidelines for immunizing your baby (also called vaccinated) vary from time to time. You can get a copy of the latest infant and adolescent immunization schedules from an agency like the Center for Disease Control and Prevention (CDC) or the American Academy of Pediatrics (AAP), or ask your child's doctor for one.

Many facilities vaccinate before the child leaves after conception. Others include vaccines once your baby is 2 months old. Anyway, most immunizations stop when he's 6 years old.

Are there reasons not to immunize my child?

Kids should NOT be vaccinated under special circumstances. For example, certain vaccines shouldn't be given to children with certain illnesses or cancer types. Some kids who shouldn't get immunized are also taking drugs that reduce the body's ability to fight infection.

 If your daughter has had a serious allergic reaction to the first shot in a series, the doctor will probably discuss the pros and cons of giving her the remainder of the series shots.

May I decide what vaccinations my child wants?

Choosing immunizations isn't a good idea. Generally, missing vaccinations isn't healthy either. This can leave your child vulnerable to potentially severe diseases otherwise avoidable.

For some children, like those who can not get certain vaccines for medical reasons, the only protection net from vaccine-preventable diseases is the immunity of people in contact with them. When vaccination levels decline, immunization-preventable diseases can become serious threats to children everywhere.

If you have questions about immunization, raise your doubts with your child's doctor. If your child falls behind the normal vaccine schedule, ask the doctor about your child's immunizations, as it's vital for their safety and well-being.

DTaP's

The DTaP vaccine is 3 in 1. D ' means Diphtheria,' T' means Tetanus, and' aP' means Pertussis. Three poor diseases your child should be immunized for. It's offered over time as a sequence of 5 shots.

Diphtheria is a heart and throat infection. It can cause heart failure and death. Often called "lockjaw," tetanus can be absorbed by dirt, rust, and grime. It can cause severe muscle spasms and death.

Pertussis (also known as "whooping cough") causes severe coughing that hinders the child's breathing, sleeping, and drinking.

It can cause pneumonia, epilepsy, brain damage, death. For about 10 years, having your child immunized while young protect against these diseases. Note, to be fully protected, your child must receive all 5 injections. Thereafter, your baby will need booster shots for these immunizations.

HBV vaccine

HBV vaccine helps prevent hepatitis B virus (HBV) disease, a liver infection that can lead to liver cancer. Hepatitis is also very infectious, easily passed from person to person. This immunization is offered as 3 or 4 shots in a sixth-month span. HBV vaccine and Hib vaccine can now be shot together, reports Lawant to Brock, scientist.

HIB vaccine

HIB is the Haemophilus type B) vaccine. This helps prevent Haemophilus influenza type b, a leading cause of serious childhood disease. It can cause meningitis, influenza, or upper respiratory infection that can cause pain and breathing difficulties. The Hib vaccine is given as 3 or 4 shots, depending on the immunization plan of your doctor.

Flu vaccine

Influenza vaccine   (also called influenza vaccine) is available by shot or nasal spray. The flu shot includes dead viruses, provided only once. Nasal-spray immunization (known as Flu-Mist) includes live but weakened viruses, often requiring two doses.

 You can't get flu from the flu shot and vaccine. Flu immunization is given in the early flu season, usually in November. Flu season usually doesn't occur until late December or January.

The flu shot is safe and effective for 6-month-old children. Nasal spray vaccine is safe for children aged 2 or older. Though, those under 2 can't get Flu-Mist. Since flu viruses vary from year to year, your child needs to get immunization every year to protect her and stay healthy. Children are more likely to have flu complications than others.

IPV vaccine

The vaccine IPV (stands for Inactivated Polio Virus) helps prevent polio, and it's been around a long time. Four times in an injection process. IPV replaced the older oral polio vaccine and is very active in eradicating polio worldwide.

Polio can cause muscle pain, one or both legs or arms paralysis, and complications. It may also paralyze muscles used to breathe and drink, resulting in death.

Meningococcal Conjugate or MCV4

The Meningococcal Conjugate Vaccine, known as MCV4, protects against 4 strains or forms of bacterial meningitis caused by bacteria meningitis. Bacterial meningitis is an infection that affects the brain and spinal cord fluid.

A chronic disease that can cause high fever, stiff neck, nausea, and headache. It can also cause more severe complications including hearing loss, brain damage, deafness, and blindness.

Kids don't get the MCV4 vaccine until age 11-12. Kids over the age of 12 who haven't had the vaccine must undergo it before starting high school, as this is a necessity.

MMR vaccine

MMR (Measles, Mumps, and Rubella) vaccine protects against these three diseases. It's given as a2-series clip. Measles can cause fever, rash, cough, sore throat, runny nose, watery eyes. It can also cause pneumonia and ear infections.

MMR vaccination makes measles very rare. Measles can also cause more serious problems, such as brain swelling and death. Mumps can cause nausea, high fever, and painful swelling of one or both main glands of saliva. Mumped children look like chipmunks with puffed-up cheeks and jaws.

Mumps can cause meningitis and, very rarely, brain swelling and death. Boys and men's testicles have been known to enlarge, which can render them unable to have children later. Rubella is like measles and is also called German measles m.

This induces nausea, rash, headache, and neck gland swelling. Rubella can also cause brain swelling and bleeding if it lasts too long. This is another infection isolated from MMR immunization. If a pregnant woman is infected with rubella, she can lose her baby or have a baby who is blind, deaf, or has trouble learning and hearing well.

The Pneumococcal Conjugate Vaccine

The Pneumococcal Conjugate Vaccine (PCV) protects against a type of bacteria commonly found in ear infections, upper respiratory infections, and pneumonia. That type of bacteria can also cause severe conditions, such as meningitis and bacteremia (bloodstream infection).

Children and children receive 4 vaccine doses in a shot sequence. Also used in older children who are at risk of pneumococcal infection.

Td Vaccine

Td vaccine is used to improve DTaP immunization. Td's Tetanus and Diphtheria. It helps prevent tetanus disease and diphtheria. Td immunization is issued when your baby is 11 and older and every 10 years for the rest of her life.

Occasionally, if there's a particularly bad wound or bone fracture, doctors can give it if the last Td shot was more than 5 years ago.

Varicella vaccine

Varicella immunization prevents varicella. Kids with chickenpox get rashes, nausea, sore throat, nasal discharge, and fatigue. Children are given once they are 12 months old or older if the baby has never had or was vaccinated for chickenpox.

Varicella vaccine is a sequence of 2 injections. Because of this vaccine, chickenpox isn't as common as before.

Safety of Immunization

You're probably concerned about immunizations, and that's a natural parental response. You want to protect your child from any harm. Remember this: vaccines are part of childhood and are important to your child's growth and development.

Keep in mind that even when your little one's sick, vaccinations can be provided. Ensure to give your child Tylenol and Motrin the first 24 hours after shooting, keep her relaxed, and take down the redness that might happen at the shot site. Another recommendation is to use an ice pack or hot, damp washcloth at the injection site. It decreases swelling and gives your child warmth. Neither makes shot time bad for her.

Explain to her it's part of staying healthy, so she doesn't have to get sick and miss out on school and sports events.

Chapter 2

The return of the old diseases: what is responsible?

For those of us who live in the sanitized security of our wonderful, practically germ-free world of hand sanitizers, wet wipes, and anti-bacterial, it is sometimes hard to imagine diseases that have all but been eradicated in the last few decades making a comeback ever.

At the start of the 20th century, U.S. life expectancy was 47 years, and today's newborns are expected to live 79 years.

More from GlobalPost: This map shows which is the deadliest infectious disease you live in, but in recent years some of the deadly diseases we thought were the stuff of history books are back with a revenge in many parts of the world— not just developing countries.

Why do preventable diseases comeback?

In the US, a recent measles outbreak was related to an increase in unvaccinated children. According to a study published in May last year by medical journal Pediatrics, up to 40% of American parents either postpone or missed vaccinations.

Those subscribing to the anti-vaccination campaign reject vaccination appeals from the Center for Disease Control (CDC), thanks in part to a now-debunked study linking vaccinations to autism.

Otherwise, the return of certain diseases is not just about parents ' choices — sometimes outbreaks arecaused by war.

In October 2013, war-ravaged Syria saw its first case of polio in 14 years as country vaccination rates fell to 52%. Aid agencies came together to combat the epidemic, vaccinating 1 million children, but around 80,000 Syrian children have not yet been vaccinated for polio, UNICEF said.

More from GlobalPost: Ukrainian children are vulnerable to a polio outbreak during war So far, only one human illness has been completely eradicated: smallpox. Today, we are facing disease outbreaks we thought we had overcome years ago.

According to the World Health Organization (WHO), this infectious and lethal disease is the leading cause of death among young people. The group reported 145,700 deaths in 2013 — which comes to 400 deaths every day or 16 deaths every hour.

A vaccine was launched in 1963, cutting measles outbreaks 99%. Today, in 17 US states, pre-school vaccination rates are below 90% and 91% nationally. That meant the re-emergence of the disease, given quick vaccine access.

 In 63 measles cases per year, the US saw an average in 2000-2007. In 2013, measles incidence doubled.

The new measles outbreak — which all started with seven people who contracted the disease during a December trip to Disneyland — has now led to nearly 200 cases of measles in the US and more than 100 in Canada.

The disease spread after an unvaccinated California woman contracted the disease while visiting the theme park and eventually made her way to the airport. According to the CDC, the virus, which persists on surfaces for up to two hours and is transmitted by sneezes and coughs, can affect 90 percent of non-immune people.

Whooping cough is another disease that has made a comeback in recent years, and the anti-vaccination campaign is not the only reason.

In 1976, the highly infectious disease, which induces severe coughing fits resulting in nausea, vomiting and even broken ribs were eradicated almost completely. There were only 1,010 infection cases back then.

CDC recorded about 28,660 cases of whooping cough in 2014—an 18 percent increase from 2013. It's as infectious as measles and more contagious than Ebola. California experienced its worst 70-year outbreak last year.

When it comes to the outbreak of pertussis, the culprit is the vaccine itself. In the 1980s, concern about the side effects of the vaccine led to the development of a new version, available throughout 1992.

The new vaccine was better but only provided temporary immunity, so doctors started prescribing a booster shot to children aged 11 or 12.

You can guess what happened next. The vaccine wore off before many kids got their booster. Others never saw the booster. And some kids got the booster but got sick instead.

"The big answer is we need a good vaccine," Mark Sawyer, University of California professor of clinical pediatrics, San Diego and federal vaccine policy advisor, told Scientific American in 2013.

"That's up to the researchers who would research what would make a better vaccine, and it's up to the pharmaceutical companies." Scarlet fever If you've read Little Women, or at least watched Friends ' episode where Joey attempts to read that, you know that the saddest moment of the book is probably the sweetest death of Beth, the youngest of the Mar.

Beth develops scarlet fever, and although she first recovers, the infection leaves her frail and eventually dies.

It's a disease that starts much like strep throat but gradually evolves into a fever, a large red rash on the skin, and a tongue of strawberries. Antibiotics are easily treated. If left untreated, it can cause serious health problems.

The UK is now seeing its worst disease outbreak in half a century, with 1,265 cases reported since early 2015.

While it won't mean any modern movie characters ' demise, it's still highly contagious. Last year, England recorded 14,000 cases of scarlet fever.

Polio It was once one of America's most dreaded illnesses, killing an average of over 35,000 people each year between the late 1940s and early 1950s, according to the CDC.

Then-President Franklin D Roosevelt bore the symptoms of this crippling disease, which in the early 1920s crippled him, almost costing him his political career.

His signature symptoms— stunted legs and paralysis— were first recorded in an ancient Egyptian victim illustration. It's a disease that people have long been struggling with.

Polio infections have dropped by over 99% since 1988. Afghanistan, Pakistan, and Nigeria are still struggling to control the spread of the deadly disease domestically and internationally.

In 2013, WHO declared the dangerously rampant spread of polio an international public health emergency after spreading nearly 60% of polio infections by adult travelers in 2013.

It can only be avoided by vaccines, and there's no cure so far.

During the 14th century it was known as the "Black Death," and back then the deadly pandemic wiped out a quarter of Europe's population.

It's a bacterial infection that enters humans by an infected rat or flea bites. Infected people grow swollen lymph nodes and ultimately pneumonia, which means coughing and sneezing can spread it.

It was largely eradicated in the developed world, but according to WHO in 2013, there were 783 reported cases and 126 deaths caused by the plague worldwide.

The bubonic plague in Madagascar killed 71 people and infected 263 since September. Last summer, areas of Yumen, a town in northwestern China, were sealed off and 30,000 people confined to their neighborhoods after a local man was killed.

Chapter 3

How Vaccinations Work

How vaccines work to stimulate the body to produce antibodies is a fascinating study regardless of your views. Not withstanding some views, vaccination has been shown to typically improve immunity to bacteria and viruses and help reduce the effects of secondary infections.

When an organism enters your body and induces infection, the body collects its defenses and battles them. It's the basic principle of how vaccines function.

Many blood cells produce what are called' antibodies,' molecules designed to attack particular germs and viruses. They bind to the bloodstream invaders, stopping them from invading other cells.

Every virus or bacterium has an individual shape, and antibodies are designed to fit that shape exactly.

This is how vaccinations work to convince the body that vaccination is a' full-blooded' attack by invading viruses or bacteria, and activate them into action to build the antibody's' memory' or' blueprint' in case of future invasion.

The white blood cells do this. You have two types of B-cells and T-cells. B cells produce antibodies while T cells have two roles. The' helper' T cells help the B cells produce the antibodies while the' killer' T cells destroy any virus or bacteria entering cells to stop them from reproducing.

Why vaccines work to induce this activity is to trick white cells into thinking the body is tainted.

The body reacts to kill the invaders in two ways: directly by the antibodies, and indirectly by killing any infected cells and preventing reproduction.

Viruses can not replicate themselves: they must use host cells for this. If the T cells continuously destroy all infected cells, antibodies will eventually kill the invaders themselves.

If the virus or bacterium is powerful and reproduces too rapidly, the host can be destroyed before it can generate enough antibodies to kill them. The fluid that develops during infection is a mixture of dead white blood cells and bacteria/virus cells destroyed by them.

If your body survives the attack, the B cells maintain a memory of the attackers ' origin and if the same viruses or bacteria ever return, it can develop antibodies rapidly and destroy the infection before it begins. This memory's activation is precisely how vaccines work.

Vaccines create the same memory benefit without enduring the disease. The disease-causing species are either destroyed or weakened and inserted into your skin. The intensity is measured so that the white cells can contain the antibodies.

That's how vaccines work to protect you from the potential disease without actually getting you sick. Vaccine strength is designed to allow this. The dead vaccine still works, but less effectively, and the result is usually not as long-lasting.

After only one or two doses, the' living' vaccines provide life-long immunity, but those' dead' and' inactivated' require multiple doses to get the right effect. Many dead vaccines even need life-long booster doses. Types are tetanus or diphtheria vaccines, normally given as Td vaccine every 10 years. The measles vaccine is a' live' vaccine.

Vaccinations do not affect your ability to combat other diseases you have not been immunized against; indeed, a German report in 2002 suggested that you are likely to have fewer illnesses in general if you have your vaccine limit.

Exactly how vaccinations function to do this is unclear, but vaccination is believed to typically improve the immune system, protecting the body against other' secondary' diseases.

Why vaccinations function to produce this secondary effect is not fully understood, but it seems that unvaccinated children may have a diminished ability to fight off a normal disease-related secondary infection, such as pneumonia, often a secondary infection in measles cases. Most deaths from measles were due to secondary pneumonia disease.

Furthermore, how vaccines work to give you immunity to the vaccinated infection is simply fooling or inducing the body to produce antibodies, and memory of their origin should the same bacteria or viruses reappear.

Chapter 2 Vaccinating or not vaccinating Everyone acknowledges that vaccination was one of the most effective public health initiatives ever taken, which remains one of the most controversial issues facing medicine today. We'll look at these controversies, trying to dissipate genuinely fallacious facts, and concentrating on real family issues.

Once the effectiveness of vaccines was known, governments rushed to make vaccinations available to the public and mandatory in many cases. When immunizations for childhood diseases emerged in the twentieth century, including diphtheria, measles, mumps, and rubella, vaccination became mandatory for public school attendance.

WHO initiated the Expanded Immunization Program in 1974. By their efforts, the world's last natural smallpox outbreak occurred in Somalia in 1977.

Governments aim to immunize as many people as possible to gain "herd immunity." Herd immunity happens when enough people are vaccinated to significantly decrease the risk of an infected person coming into contact.

Sadly, though finding vaccines was likely one of the most important steps in eradicating the disease (along with sanitation and antibiotics), safety issues associated with vaccine administration have been and remain.

Two lots of polio vaccine contained the live virus in 1955, causing polio outbreak. A paper was published in the 1970s, linking pertussis vaccination to permanent brain damage.

The subsequent boycott of vaccines and litigation forced vaccine manufacturers out of business, causing shortages and rapidly increasing disease incidence. The claim was later disproved, but the dispute led to the development of the National Vaccine Information

Office, the National Vaccine Injury Act, which gives manufacturers some liability protection, and the National Vaccine Injury Compensation Program, which offers monetary compensation when a vaccine is found to have a deleterious effect.

There was a concern in 1976 that the swine flu outbreak could cause an epidemic as devastating as the 1918 flu epidemic which killed 50,000,000 people worldwide.

 The swine flu vaccine was rushed to the public without proper screening, leading to about 500 cases of Guillain-Barré syndrome until program termination.

Vaccines, like any medication or foreign material entering the body, can cause allergic reactions, often due to adjuvants, i.e. substances used by the vaccine as a medium of administration.

 Localized swelling, fever, vomiting and more side effects are often associated with injections.

Beyond the concern about individual vaccination issues as mentioned above, there is a large minority of people who believe the growing rates of autism and learning disabilities in the U.S. is linked to their compulsory immunization program.

Some work has been done on both sides of the issue, and there is no conclusive evidence to support or refute these views.

Autism is a developmental disorder that impairs social behaviors and relationships. Such habits usually occur at about eighteen months. Most vaccines are issued on a schedule starting at age 2 months, raising debate as to whether immunizations cause autism.

Historical review shows that autism prevalence rose at about the time the U.S. MMR vaccine was introduced. Nevertheless, autism awareness as a separate condition grew concurrently. British autism didn't increase after MMR was implemented there.

Thimerosal, organic mercury, was historically used as a vaccine element. Fears of a mercury-autism connection prompted the Institute of Medicine to demand vaccine elimination of thimerosal as a precautionary measure. This change, not based on scientific evidence, justified these fears. The current scientific consensus is that thimerosal induces or worsens autism; almost all vaccines eliminated this element by 1999.

Ultimately, vaccines have improved the lives of billions of people worldwide, eradicating or limiting most diseases to small, manageable outbreaks.

To vaccinate proponents invoke the following points.

Getting vaccinated protects the patient and community; promoting the public good is an obligation to live in a society.

While most vaccine advocates agree that there may be specific cases where vaccination is not required, they point out that if vaccines weaken the immune system, there should be a lower infection rate following immunization. A 2001 survey of over 800,000 children in Denmark found no correlation.

It is not fair to subject vaccinated children, particularly those who have been vaccinated because their medical conditions indicate that the vaccine would have serious negative effects, to the risk of getting the disease from those who choose not to be vaccinated (because most vaccines are not 100% effective).

 Kids who are not vaccinated with MMR (Mumps, Measles, and Rubella) are 35 times more likely to get major diseases. Varicella can cause hospitalization and/or death. Polio vaccination is essential as polio is still present in developing countries.

Such diseases are rare due to high immunization. When people choose to avoid vaccinating, pathogens can recover, as shown by research in other countries.

There is still no credible evidence of the autism-vaccination connection. This stance is sponsored by the World Health Organization, CDC, AMA, and the American Pediatrics Academy.

Although vaccines are spectacularly effective in the macro sense, on a person-by-person basis, vaccines may cause mild to severe side effects and/or permanent and crippling harm. There is a fundamental belief that the state can not pressure people to submit to unnecessary medical interventions.

As a result, some people, especially parents of vaccine-age children, support NOT TO VACCINATE and use the following reasons :-

That person or family has the right to make free choices about invasive medical procedures. Recognizing the macro value of vaccination, each person or family need the freedom to assess their circumstance, particularly as regards vulnerabilities, and then choose the best course of action for individuals.

Vaccines are actively promoted by manufacturers ' profit motive. If immunization cases go to court, vaccine companies will supply "bought" experts to plead their case.

The U.S. Vaccine Compensation Program paid nearly 2,000 damages (over $1.2 billion) for vaccine harm, including a recent case where the court found that multiple immunizations induced autism symptoms.

 Kids with autoimmune diseases are at higher risk of severe side effects from vaccines and should be able to participate.

The Vaccine Adverse Event Reporting System (VAERS), a government-run system that collects data on vaccine-related adverse events, receives over 1,000 reports each month, measured at about 10% of actual events.

Immunization of hepatitis B is not worthwhile-the disease does not even affect children (less than 1% of all confirmed patients are under the age of 15) yet it carries the risk of adverse effects, including death.

For less dangerous diseases like measles and chickenpox, natural immunity is preferred because it is 100% successful.

Vaccines contain recognized toxins such as aluminum and thimerosal.

MMR vaccine side effects are similar to disease and can be serious. Varicella side effects are similar to infection; naturally acquired disease offers immunity for life, vaccine requires boosters.

Polio vaccination is unnecessary because wild polio hasn't happened in the United States for 20 years. Such illnesses are so rare that it's highly unlikely anybody will develop them anymore.

While the link between increased autism and increased vaccination may not be causal, it may still be causal. Vaccinations should not be necessary.

Not surprisingly, there are strong feelings on both sides of this issue, fuelled by huge amounts of misinformation on the Internet. While is this problem middle ground or any solutions?

The approach is more and better multi-faceted analysis. We want solutions for autism and vaccines. Equally important is to work into new and better ways to produce vaccines to be more efficient and less likely to create adverse events in specific individuals.

The middle ground is likely represented by the United States and Canada, maintaining an extremely high level of vaccination and low levels of preventable diseases, but at the same time providing opportunities for individuals in most situations to be excluded from the need for religious or medical vaccination.

That balance helps the majority of the population to be well covered while still allowing people the freedom to choose freely.

Should you vaccinate children?

Will you vaccinate your kids? This is a problem every parent faces almost as soon as their child is born because the first vaccine is given shortly after birth (HepB) according to the CDC vaccination schedule.

It can sometimes be a controversial topic, so let me completely announce that anything in the future is purely my opinion on my children's vaccinations.

I've already vaccinated and will continue to vaccinate both of my boys because I heard something that stuck with me during my short nursing stay.

"Why would you keep taking your child to a doctor you don't trust?" What is this about vaccination? I fully trust everything my boy's doctor believes in and he, like most, believes in vaccinating his patients entirely.

There's no definitive answer to this question because the decision lies solely with the family, so I'll just go over some vaccination pros and cons as well as some common myths surrounding vaccination.

Vaccines Bottom line, vaccines can save your child's life. Some diseases your baby will be vaccinated against under the CDC vaccination schedule may be deadly. For example, the MMR vaccine protects against Measles, Mumps, and Rubella that can all be deadly.

Vaccination can save your family time and money. We all know that medical bills are costly, particularly if you have heavy co-paid coverage, and vaccinating your kids could save you the exorbitant amount of money you'd spend on medical bills if your kid came down with any of the diseases the current vaccination schedule vaccinates against.

Vaccination prevents future generations. By vaccination, diseases that once infected and killed thousands of people are now virtually eliminated or near extinction. For example, the last cases of naturally occurring U.S. paralytic Polio were in 1979. This is thanks to the vaccine miracle, and parents continue to trust their children's doctor!

Vaccinations are safe and efficient. We all know it's tough to watch our kids get vaccines, but if you equate that to what they'd go through if they catch any of the diseases they're safe from, it's nothing.

Cons Vaccinations can cause discomfort. Let's face it, shots don't feel good, especially for kids. Although seeing your kids scream and kick from vaccinations can be difficult, it's a huge difference from how you'd feel if your baby had one of the diseases they're vaccinated for.

Side effects. Many, if not all, compulsory vaccinations can cause mild side effects that may include a sore injection site or low-grade fever. Such side effects will subside after a few days, but can still be frustrating for younger kids.

The government controls the vaccine decision. I agree that the decision to vaccinate or not should be made solely by the parents, but in most cases, it is not because the entry requirements for public schools in most states require that your child be vaccinated.

However, the decision to vaccinate rests solely on the mother, and although I have fully vaccinated all my children and will continue to do so, I fully respect the decision of anyone not to vaccinate.

Common myths about vaccination Myth 1: vaccination causes autism This myth emerged in 1997 when a British surgeon named Andrew Wakefield published an article. A medical journal, The Lancet, published an article linking children's increased chance of autism to a particular vaccine, Measles, Mumps, and Rubella (MMR).

The good news is that this report has since been debunked due to multiple procedural errors, ethical breaches and financial conflicts of interest (sounds like a kickback contract to me!). Dr. Wakefield has lost his medical license, withdrawing the article from The Lancet.

The bad news is that the medical community took this study very seriously, leading to many other major studies eventually leading to the discovery that there was no real link between any vaccine and the risk of children having autism from administering the vaccine.

The true cause of autism remains a mystery, but to disprove this theory, numerous studies have reported autism symptoms in children well before they receive the MMR vaccine.

Myth 2: Children's immune systems can't handle so many vaccines Children are, in most situations, much more resilient than most parents think (including myself), which also relates to their immune systems.

For example, based on the number of antibodies in an infant's blood, they would be able to respond to around 10,000 vaccines at once.

The CDC recommends 14 planned vaccinations, and even if a baby got all these vaccines at once, it would only use about 0.1% of their immune system (not to mention that I would never be able to sit through my babies having 14 injections at once!).

The idea that a child's immune system "can't handle" vaccines is purely theoretical because scientists believe an "immune system power."

Myth 3: Vaccinating your baby is not worth the risk As a mother, I can fully understand wanting the best for your child and even when it comes to giving my boys Tylenol, I try to avoid it unless necessary, but when it comes to vaccines, children have been vaccinated safely for a long time, so I am personally assured that there are no quantifiable risks.

When it comes to immediate vaccine risk, talking of serious side effects and allergic reactions, the occurrence of death is so low that it can not even be measured.

For example, around 1990-1992, only one death confirmed to the CDC was caused directly from a vaccine. The odds of a vaccine-related severe allergic reaction are about one in every one to two million injections.

Myth 4: Why vaccinate for diseases/infections no longer around?

I heard this one a lot, "Why should I vaccinate my kids for diseases that haven't existed for years?"

What they don't know is that as long as a large portion of a population is immunized against a contagious disease due to Population Immunity, many members of that community will be safe against that infection because there is very little chance for an outbreak.

The CDC warns that international travel is growing rapidly, so even if a disease is not a concern in the United States, it can very well be widespread in another country. If a person carries a disease from another state, anyone who has not been vaccinated will have a much greater risk of contracting the disease.

Chapter 4

Vaccines -Why Anxiety Sells

It's curious how a vaccine debate can get heated and sometimes even aggressive. Would the same controversy rage over an antibiotic or antihypertensive treatment if the medication caused harm?

 When it becomes clear that a drug like Vioxx hurt thousands, it is removed from the market. We stop using drugs until proven safe. And we're investigating.

Not with vaccination. Vaccines are marketed with fanfare until they are scientifically shown to affect most people.

The thousands of individuals who suffer from vaccine reactions in proportion to the millions vaccinated are not considered to be mathematically important.

However, the more than $1billion charged to vaccine-injured people shows that security isn't all it's claimed to be. Why the double standard?

Vaccination is founded on a "belief system." We believe that vaccines are safe; we believe that vaccinations are vital for health; we believe stories that vaccines are solely responsible for removing smallpox and polio.

And we want to trust that our doctors have read all available vaccine information— pro and con— or told us the full truth about vaccines.

Belief, however, is based on faith, not inherently reality. They want to assume, for instance, that vaccinating our kids can prevent them from getting sick with measles or chickenpox. Though, there's plenty of data showing that's not so.

Why is the current belief— and trust— in vaccines almost desperate to defend? The public's view of the disease appears close to our current view of terrorism: sporadic, potentially deadly attacks.

Press hawks this view of childhood disease and vaccine need. Pharma sells, physicians, move it, and educational institutions reinforce it. They keep selling it, because they purchase it most readily, without a doubt.

There is an attitude of "just in case" and "better than sorry" when it comes to vaccination and illness for children. * After nearly 200 years of use, fear still sells vaccination.

What do we know about vaccines? A study of literature and CDC reports reveals:

1. Vaccine safety studies were relatively small, with only healthy children.

Nevertheless, when a vaccine trial is completed, ALL children receive vaccines regardless of their fitness, family history, or genetics.

2. Safety studies were short. Most clinical trials track 21 days for side effects, sometimes only 5 days. Complications of the immune system can take months.

The arbitrary date, set by the FDA, precludes associating vaccinations with chronic health conditions. "Free" is a classification with limited information.

3. Vaccine safety trials do not use a real placebo. The placebo-controlled trial is one of the Gold Standards for medical research. One group of patients receives an inert substance, such as a sugar pill, a placebo, while the treatment group receives the new drug.

The data were evaluated to compare the number of side effects in those given the drug to the number of side effects in those given placebo. Nevertheless, the "placebo" used in vaccine research is not an inert material like sterile water; another vaccine. Inert, sterile water does not react; as vaccine replacement does.

If both baby classes in a trial have the same number of reactions, the study reports that the vaccine "is as healthy as placebo."

4. Vaccine-induced antibodies are not safe. Nonetheless, the respected paper, Vaccine stated it simply"... it is understood that antigen-specific titers do not correlate with safety in many cases." Vaccination was accepted as secure, efficient and protective. The shots can be characterized as a medical "sacred cows," by default, "a medical procedure that is unreasonably immune to criticism." The strong response is a reaction to a suggestion that the "cow" should be "sacrificed."

Once Copernicus insisted that the moon, not the earth, was the center of the solar system, this went against pagan philosophical and religious values.

Although two other contemporary Italian thinkers, Galileo and Bruno, followed the Copernican theory, their remarks were considered blasphemous. Before the Inquisition, Bruno was tried, condemned and burned in 1600.

Thirty years later, Galileo was brought forward and forced to renounce his views under threat of torture and death before his "Betters." Even after confession, he was sentenced to jail for the remaining days.

The more one explores vaccination and discusses the adverse effects that have been linked to vaccines, the more one becomes a Copernican heretic, which can have deadly consequences. I've spent over 8,000 hours revealing the truth about vaccines.

If the result of this investigation and disclosure is to be called a heretic, I'm in a wonderful company.

Chapter 5

What do vaccines contain?

Having the infection you receive the vaccine, such as mumps, may potentially be a blessing to the infected and give the illness true immunity. This may account for some of the disease-preventing effects of vaccines in a small number of vaccinated individuals.

However, the vast majority of the vaccinated population is not ill. If so, vaccination may potentially have some benefit.

However, if an adjuvant such as aluminum or squalene is introduced to the vaccine now standard of most vaccinations, it can cause the immune system to overreact to the presence of the organism against which you are being vaccinated.

In such times, the human body becomes powerless against foreign material, overcome by antigens and the resulting immune system overreaction.

This often contributes to deteriorating symptoms (thimerosal, linked to neurological damage in the brain, is among the most frequently released agents via vaccines), debilitating side effects, and even life-threatening conditions.

Given documented evidence linking vaccination with disease and injury, modern medicine maintains vaccinations are a form of' health insurance.' But just so you know your facts, here's a brief look at what they involve.

Antigen: The disease-causing microorganism or pathogen against which immunity is sought is the crux of any vaccine.

Preservatives: Preservatives are used to improve a vaccine's shelf-life, stopping bacteria and fungi from destroying it. In the US, the FDA approves three preservatives: phenol,2-phenoxyethanol, and thimerosal.

Adjuvants: Adjuvants improve the immune response of the body immediately after the vaccine. While highly dangerous and known to cause cytokine storms which lead to rapid death, pharmaceutical companies continue to use adjuvants as vaccine boosters.

Another compelling reason for using adjuvants is that these chemicals, by turbo-charging vaccines, allow drug makers to use less of the antigen in each dose to produce more doses. Do the math: more doses means more income.

Aluminum salts are the adjuvants used most by drug manufacturers. These include aluminum phosphate, aluminum hydroxide, aluminum hydroxyphosphate sulfate, and aluminum aluminum aluminum sulfate.

Before recently, aluminum salts were the only adjuvant vaccine-makers permitted to use in the US. Nevertheless, with the FDA playing with the idea of allowing squalene as an adjuvant, there is growing concern that this drug, playing havoc with veterans of the US Gulf War, maybe approved for widespread use in the US.

Additives or Stabilizing Agents: Stabilizing agents protect vaccines from damage or loss of effectiveness under conditions such as freezing and heat. These often stop antigens from sticking to the side of the vaccine vial and removing vaccine components.

Popular additives include sugars such as sucrose and lactose; amino acids such as glycine, monosodium glutamate; and proteins such as gelatin or albumin from human serum.

Concerns about these additives center around the use of gelatin, human serum albumin and bovine material, particularly cows. Although gelatin can precipitate hypersensitivity reactions, human serum albumin (derived from dead human fetuses) may introduce pathogens into the body.

Bovine Spongiform Encephalopathy and' mad cow disease' in England in the 1980s concentrated on content obtained from cattle.

Residual agents: residual agents are used during processing to inactivate the live pathogen and to cultivate the virus. We are eventually excluded from the vaccine, or at least that's what vaccine-makers say.

Residual agents include bovine serum (a common agent used in cell cultures to develop the virus); formaldehyde (used as an inactivating agent); and antibiotics such as neomycin, streptomycin, and polymyxin B to prevent bacterial contamination.

Animal Products: In vaccine manufacturing, animal products are most commonly used as the medium in which the virus grows and grows. They serve two essential functions: they provide the pathogen with nutrients and provide cell lines that enable it to multiply to make millions of doses sold commercially.

Animals usually used to produce vaccines are monkeys, goats, horses, chickens, pigs and sometimes dogs and rabbits.

Human Products: Human fetal cells (human diploid cells) split continuously, allowing cell lines to replicate a virus. The rubella virus, for instance, grows in human tissue culture as the virus can not infect animals.

Upon growing a virus, the pathogen is removed when extracting it from the growth culture. Traces of plant genetic material, however, remain in the vaccine.

That's a true, ever-present danger. If the host animal or person is infected, secondary pathogens may be transmitted during vaccination.

That's exactly what happened when Simian Vacuolating Virus 40 or SV40 later found the polio vaccine, developed in monkey kidney cells.

Looking at the large element categories in vaccines, here is a list of some toxic agents (with reported side effects) used in their development.

Oil Adjuvants: A neurotoxin related to Alzheimer's disease and seizures. Arthritis Formaldehyde: A carcinogenic agent used as an embalming fluid Ethylene Glycol: Antifreeze commonly used in car engines Triton X100: A detergent Glycerin: Can damage internal organs such as lungs, liver and kidneys and gastrointestinal tract Monosodium glutamate (MSG): According to the FDA, MSG Symptom Complex or MSG side effects can result in numbness, burning glutamate (MSG)

Indeed, studies have shown that MSG can cause arrhythmia, atrial fibrillation, tachycardia, rapid heartbeat, palpitations, sluggish heartbeat, angina, severe rise or drop in blood pressure, swelling, diarrhea, nausea / vomiting, cramps of the stomach, rectal bleeding, bloating, flu-like pain, joint pain, stiffness, depression, mood swings, rabies, migraine headache, dizziness etc.

Phenol and carbolic acid: a lethal toxin used as a disinfectant in household and industrial products and dye thimerosal (mercury derivative): a poisonous heavy metal used as a preservative.

Aluminum: a metallic component which, besides destroying the brain in infants, can also predispose adults to neurological problems such as Alzheimer's and Polysorbate 80 (Tween80TM) dementia: an emulsifier that can cause severe allergic reactions, including anaphylaxis.

Furthermore, according to a Slovak rat study published in the 1993 journal Food and Chemical Toxicology, Tween80 could contribute to infertility. Tween 80 increased rat maturation, extended the estrous cycle, decreased the weight of the uterus and ovaries, and caused damage to the uterus lining suggesting persistent estrogenic stimulation.

All this makes me wonder why so many millions of people started suffering from diseases that are identified as side effects of these toxins after widespread vaccinations have been implemented into modern societies. Most of these diseases were almost unheard of before vaccine-mania started.

Chapter 6

Do we give our children too many vaccines?

Families are particularly concerned about the number of vaccines children currently receive. Government schools allow children to complete the required vaccines before enrolling in college.

The list of vaccinations needed continues to rise along with costs. The amount of vaccinations poses concerns about safety and explanations for many vaccines.

To put the situation in perspective, children received a single vaccine for smallpox around 100 years ago. Through time, vaccine numbers increased to five, around forty-five years ago.

 Such five vaccines were diphtheria, pertussis, tetanus, measles, and smallpox. In the past forty years, the number doubles where today's kids receive 11 daily vaccines. Many of the vaccines were multiple-shot.

Increasing vaccine costs In the early 1980s, the cost of immunizing a child with the necessary vaccines was $75-$100. Not only has the number of vaccines doubled, but the price has also tripled.

The cost of obtaining the prescribed vaccines is about $1,250. Even with inflation, cost increases are drastic. The price would rise for teenage girls. Vaccination which currently protects against cervical cancer costs about $360 for a three-dose collection, bringing the vaccine total to about $1600.

Although the number of shots has been decreased, the combination shots make it difficult to track that shot children encounter when side effects occur.

The number of Antigens Children are exposed to many of these vaccines are for multiple antigens due to the increased expense. (An antigen is a molecule that causes the immune system to produce chemical substances called' anti-bodies' when injected into your body.

Such antibodies are programmed to either destroy or neutralize any substance they consider a' threat'.) Combination shots increase the cost of vaccines. Another explanation for combination shots is an attempt to decrease the number of physical doses the child receives.

The number of chemicals pumped into children's developing bodies is incredible. When a woman takes all doses of all necessary vaccines, the number of antigens received in 45 shots is 156. Boys, in about 42 doses, receive 144 vaccine antigens.

Think about it for a moment. Following the vaccine schedule, you inject 144-156 alien chemicals into your developing body. Through vaccines, these substances are injected into the bloodstream and bypass the body's natural defenses.

You may find it stupid to take your child to 150 different chemical plants to be exposed to these chemicals, but when you obey the schedule, you take similar action.

If your child is susceptible or allergic to many foreign chemicals, adding this many chemicals in such a short period asks for trouble.

The government recommends multiple vaccines. The vaccines needed include hepatitis A and B; inactivated poliovirus (IPV); rotavirus; Haemophilus influenzae Type B (Hib); measles, mumps, rubella (MMR); pneumococcal conjugate (PCV); varicella (chickenpox); influenza; and diphtheria, tetanus and acellular pertussis (DTaP).

Furthermore, tetanus-diphtheria and acellular pertussis vaccine and meningitis vaccine (MCV4) are available for those entering high school.

Studies reported reactions to pertussis and chickenpox vaccines. The risk is that many of those vaccinated develop shingles within 10 years of vaccination.

Vaccination is one of the 20th century's ten greatest achievements in public health. Nevertheless, it does not take an advanced degree in science to understand that public health accolades, praising high vaccination rates and low infection rates, have resulted in severe health consequences worldwide.

These include immune responses to vaccine ingredients. Vaccine products seem to play a significant role in today's health problems.

Often, vaccine additives cause problems rather than the vaccines themselves. Gelatin, one of many ingredients was recorded.

Allergies and asthma. Vaccines known to contain gelatin include chickenpox, MMR, Boostrix (a juvenile pertussis booster), Tripedia (DTaP) and Zostrix, the adult shingle vaccine.

Another dangerous additive, formaldehyde. It's used to inactivate many vaccine bacteria. Often found to disrupt the immune system's normal function. Although the CDC page downplays formaldehyde exposure and risk, the National Cancer Institute describes it as' known human carcinogen.'

Besides being a preservative for lab samples, formaldehyde can cause watery eyes, burning eye and throat sensations, vomiting, breathing difficulties, and asthma attacks. The material is listed as dangerous on eight federal regulatory lists.

With the new vaccine, children receive over 10 times the required safe doses. Formaldehyde-including DTaP, measles, and influenza vaccines.

Another common ingredient, MSG. Use MSG to' stabilize' vaccines. MSG is often used as a flavor enhancer but agitates the neural system in some populations. Some find MSG to be an excitotoxin as it agitates and' excites' the nervous system.

Many vaccines do produce egg-proteins. Although government sites downplay the potential reaction, people allergic to egg proteins that respond to these substances.

Many contaminants in many vaccines are adjuvants. These are additives used to improve vaccine drugs ' potency.

Adjuvates intensify vaccine effects. Several forms of chemicals are used to improve vaccine potency. Aluminum salt variations are often used in human-based vaccines.

Occasionally vaccines contain oil-based adjuvates. Another controversial is squalene. Squalene activates fast auto-immune antibodies response. In many circles, Squalene is controversial. No US-produced vaccines, according to CDC, contain squalene.

"There is no squalene in an FDA-approved vaccine in the US. There is no squalene in any form of seasonal flu vaccine or H1N1 vaccine."-Patricia El-Hinnawy It contradicts vaccine manufacturers ' claims. One GlaxoSmithKline spokesman says his vaccines have squalene.

"A novel aspect of the two H1N1 vaccines being produced by Novartis and GlaxoSmithKline is the introduction of squalene-containing adjuvants to improve immunogenicity and significantly reduce the amount of viral antigen required, resulting in much faster development of targeted vaccine quantities."

Meryl Nass, MD With all the debate, parents should consider the old Latin phrase. You need to examine yourself and seek the medical information you trust.

The 2007 sales figures for preventive vaccines amounted to $16.3bn. This is an improvement from 2006's $11.7 billion. With many vaccines approved by governments, the risk of declining sales is small. The portion of these figures for childhood vaccinations was $8bn.

Chapter 7

The Law on Forced Vaccination

One State, in particular, Massachusetts, has concentrated on its Pandemic Response Act, which now requires the governor to declare a state of emergency and view common citizens as victims of violence if they do not agree to forced vaccination.

Notwithstanding vociferous opposition from civil liberties groups, parents ' organizations, lawyers, consumer groups and another protesting, concerned and enlightened people, the House of Representatives gave the bill a resounding thumbs-up in August 2009.

Never before had any American state-approved police intervention in healthcare and vaccination.

This bill scandalously allows police to search homes physically without a warrant, violently quarantine residents, remove children from their homes and vaccinate them against their own will and that of their parents, and encourage the state governor to impose martial law.

Of course, ordinary people refusing these efforts "in the name of public health" can be incarcerated without charges or jury.

Regarding the law, when a pandemic is announced, people seem to have little choice but to report to the state or face criminal charges. And the government, as it were, follows the WHO's 194-signatory diktats.

It means that, should their respective governments so choose, the populations of 194 countries might theoretically be subject to policies like those introduced in Massachusetts!

Such unexplained steps, known by many as' Gestapo tactics,' have sparked a debate on what recourse people have when faced with such tyranny.

Several people, parents, and others have developed groups that bring the issue of anti-vaccination to the leaders of their country, hoping persuasive methods would persuade their political representatives not to use coercive tactics against the public.

Nevertheless, seeing mass vaccines from a historical perspective is an uphill task. Public or compulsory vaccination policy dates back to the 19th century when smallpox was widespread. Even then, it evoked public backlash, with some states seeking to abolish these stringent laws.

The 19th-century transition saw a landmark case that became the touchstone for all U.S. public health legislation-the Jacobson vs. Massachusetts case. In 1905, the U.S.

Supreme Court dismissed an argument that compulsory vaccines violated every citizen's right to care for their safety.

The court revoked the claimant's right to public safety. Therefore, the court set the tone for state vaccination laws, and since then the federal authorities have granted that state the power to make and enforce its vaccination laws.

The Supreme Court has always tended to help the states in numerous cases against forced vaccination, rendering the cause of people much more difficult.

However, each state usually follows federal authorities ' directives, which in turn obey the CDC's agenda, which in turn is considered to be part of pharmaceutical companies. That's a vicious cycle.

The 1960s, due to massive measles outbreaks, introduced much tighter legal restrictions. There was no looking back after this. Vaccine manufacturers developed older and newer vaccines and, potentially, disease vaccines.

And it was there. Vaccine manufacturers find a captive market for their toxic formulations— children. By whipping up fear in the minds of anxious and uninformed parents, they began pushing their goods through the school agenda, beginning with playschool!

Not surprisingly, the number of vaccines prescribed for babies and children has increased over the years.

That state has its vaccination laws regarding what vaccinations should be given and at what age and stage in a school-going child's life. And this public threat won't escape if you opt-out of the program.

The truth is, parents who refuse to vaccinate their children should remove their wards from schools. On the other hand, parents who don't send their children to school infringe state truancy rules!

But every person possesses other rights, even against forced vaccination. Yes, there are certain rules and regulations to be enforced by public health agencies, again within the law.

Right to Informed Consent: No person may be required to vaccinate. He or she must be aware of the potential risks, complications, and side effects associated with the vaccine and other warning material made public by health authorities such as CDC and FDA. Such data must be made available before any vaccine is administered.

The Right to Informed Consent is rooted in the 1986 National Childhood Vaccine Injury Act, which mandates all physicians and other vaccine suppliers to provide informed vaccination data to parents before they are vaccinated.

It is this privilege that people and parents are deliberately robbed for mass school vaccination drives. The fear-mongering, mass hysteria, and emotionally manipulative methods embraced by the forces which scare people into' consenting' to vaccination.

In these cases, people are unlikely to receive a vaccine; they are more likely to take' protective action.'

Exemptions: All 50 American states require vaccine plans for children seeking entry to a different school and college grades. While the number and type of vaccines vary from state to state, all state-licensed educational institutions have specific vaccination laws.

But did you know that parents on medical grounds could refuse to send coercive diktats? For example, if your child has a history of adverse reactions to earlier vaccination attempts, you might seek medical exemption from further vaccination.

Different states require different applicants. While some states allow a simple written letter from a family physician outlining reasons for a medical exemption, others reserve the right to review and even circumvent it.

The second reason for seeking an exemption is religious, as some religions do not allow vaccination or any form of invasive medical treatment. While some states only interpret the word ' religious beliefs' loosely, others allow the applicant to belong to a specific religious faith category.

Also, while some need a letter of recommendation from the applicant's religious leader, others are tougher and rely on an affidavit.

Exemption from compulsory vaccination is embedded in the U.S. Constitution's First Amendment, which grants every person the right to freely exercise their faith.

To revoke this right and enforce vaccination, the government must show "compelling state interest," which could be the spread of communicable diseases.

Ironically, religious groups like the Amish who practice this constitutional right do not allow their families to vaccinate and do not have communicable diseases or autistic children. This makes much sense to me.

The third type of exclusion is a religious exemption, which represents the personal beliefs of an individual prohibiting vaccination.

This is the most arbitrary of the three types of exceptions, but let me explain what happens when parents come together to launch a concerted and coordinated fight for their rights.

It may have taken seven long years in Texas and two in Arkansas, but people in both states finally gained the constitutional right to exercise vaccine exemptions for conscientious, political and religious beliefs.

Miffed by this hard-fought win, federal health officials are gradually lobbying state legislators to revoke the waiver. By 2010, 48 out of 50 US states permit religious exemption while 18 allow personal, philosophical or conscientious exemption from vaccination.

Of course, to obtain an exemption is easier said than done as parents should comply with various formalities, let alone be given one. Not surprisingly, more and more people use this term to work around compulsory vaccinations. Not surprisingly, even on medical and religious grounds, obtaining exemptions has become increasingly difficult.

The first step in stopping the government from entering the body is to educate yourself on vaccination. As mentioned above, all states have vaccination laws, which differ between states.

Educate yourself on state laws so you can make an informed choice for you and your family. As more and more people are waking up to traditional medicine's harmful effects, various forums and pressure groups are gathering to demand citizens ' rights. Joining one of these sites may be a good idea.

Here's an example of what internet spending a few minutes can show. For example, a quick search will reveal that while the American Academy of Pediatrics and the CDC recommend that all children receive the MMR (measles, mumps, rubella), the legislation in your state that mandate that children be vaccinated against measles and rubella only.

Vaccination is becoming more common in different aspects of life and can affect important adoption choices and decisions, child custody agreements during divorce proceedings, health insurance, and government programs access, medical care and immigration.

In a disturbing trend, further highlighting Big Pharma's stranglehold on government and the medical profession, pediatricians have started to refuse to offer medical treatment for children who have not met all vaccination requirements under the law.

Hospitals have even reported parents to child social services organizations for their failure or inability to vaccinate their children. As ridiculous as it is, it's the bitter truth. Therefore, educating yourself on the rules is more important than ever.

Soldiers: Army soldiers, especially recruits, are a favorite vaccine testing ground in mass immunization programs. Military troops should send vaccines in the name of preparation for battle.

 All men and women have little alternative but constant treatments to' protect' them from bio-toxins like smallpox, anthrax, ricin and other diseases.

Many soldiers died from the frequently untested chemicals in these experimental vaccines, and others were severely sick.

 Like women involved in unconscious ultrasound tests, in massive drug trials, soldiers are guinea pigs. How else could the pharmaceutical industry safely check human poisons?

Sadly, in the armed forces, you have few civil rights. Therefore, soldiers can not deny vaccination. Those who deny their shots face martial court and detention, or at least dishonorable discharge.

Common side effects of U.S. soldiers ' over one million vaccines have included joint pain, extreme fatigue, and memory loss. One example is the anthrax vaccine provided to Gulf War veterans in the Middle East war of 1992.

Health or religious exceptions are allowed, however, exemptions must be obtained before enlisting. Once the candidate enlists with the armed forces, he/she pretty much signs over his / her body to the U.S. Defense Department, which has been repeatedly accused of human experimentation.

Chapter 8

The development of a needle-free vaccination delivery system has been identified by the Grand Challenges in Global Health (GCGH) initiative described the implementation of a needle-free vaccination program as one of the major challenges facing global health care today.

Every day healthcare requires millions of needles and syringes. The World Health Organization (WHO) predicts an annual infusion of 12 billion. Only about 5% are used for immunization and infectious disease prevention vaccines.

While vaccines have saved lives over the years, some obstacles must be overcome. One is using needles or "sharps" to administer vaccines.

According to Myron Levine of the Center for Vaccine Development, University of Maryland School of Medicine and member of the Global Alliance for Vaccines and Immunization (GAVI).

Three fundamental themes remain consistent worldwide: first, high immunization coverage of target populations generally has to be achieved for full public health impact; second, no existing vaccines are administered equally; A large fraction of our population is afraid of needles, possibly due to previous bad experiences.

The disadvantages of needle delivery of vaccine include:

1. Most patients at the vaccine delivery end are very young children under the age of two, and needle pricks in this patient population can cause pain and distress. Needles can also cause injection site pain long after the shot is applied.

(2) Non-compliance. The World Health Organization's Expanded Immunization Initiative (EPI) recommended six basic infant vaccines in developing countries:

diphtheria, pertussis and tetanus toxoids (DPT), Calmette-Guerin Bacillus (BCG), and polio and measles attenuated. For developed countries like the US, health authorities need more vaccines. Nevertheless, for the so-called "herd immunity" to work, several percents of the population must follow the vaccination schedule.

(3) Security. Vaccination with needles creates hazardous infectious waste that poses serious threats to patients and healthcare professionals. Reusing unsterilized needles has encouraged blood-borne diseases such as HIV and hepatitis.

(4) Speed, performance. Recently, the risks of bioterrorism and pandemic flu have highlighted the need to provide fast, simple and secure vaccines to the masses if the need arises. Vaccination with syringes and needles was certainly not built for these cases.

(5) Cost-efficient logistics. Eliminating syringes and needles will make vaccines cheaper and more accessible in less-developed countries. It must be delivered and processed for vaccination purposes. Refrigerate injectable vaccines during travel.

While needle-free delivery systems exist for many medications, vaccines are difficult because they typically consist of large molecules that can not be distributed transdermally easily. In a review article, Myron Levine outlined different methods for delivering needle-free vaccines.

(1) Vaccines from mucosal surfaces. While theoretically possible, this method of delivery was not caught except perhaps by using the nasal spray.

(2) Vaccines nasal. Similar pill vaccines can be given orally. The oral polio vaccine has long been around. That path can provide certain vaccinations, including certain forms of cholera vaccines and modern rotavirus vaccines.

This delivery method, however, poses some issues for very young infants who may not be able to swallow properly and whose digestive system may not be able to withstand vaccine effects.

(3) Vaccines nasal. The respiratory tract nasal vaccine is a popular alternative to the flu shot. FluMist's nasal spray, made from the live, attenuated, cold-adapted vaccine, has

been approved by the FDA and is administered through the nostrils using a single-use spray system.

(4) Aerosol vaccine, which has been evaluated for the measles vaccine as an alternative to nasal spray and can be used with liquid aerosol or dry control for mass immunization.

(5) Percutaneous jet-injection needle-free. It operates by propelling fluid under high pressure through a tiny skin pore. The fluid is then transferred to the dermis and tissues and muscles.

Several dose injectors are available, making this method of delivery fast and practical for mass immunization. Nonetheless, it has the downside of a high incidence of local annoyance at the vaccination site and the risk of infectious disease transmission.

(6) Transcutaneous availability. This is commonly called "vaccine mask" and is administered through the body. Upon pre-hydration, the adhesive patch is applied directly to the body.

The occlusive patch renders vaccine-permeable hair. Langerhans cells located in the skin's upper layer (epidermis) then take up the cutaneously added antigens, allowing the immune-processing cells to migrate to the lymph nodes.

Many biotech companies have invested millions of dollars in designing, researching and finalizing various forms of needle-free delivery systems for all kinds of drugs, not just vaccines. At this juncture, the most effective needle-free vaccine programs are transcutaneous immunization (TCI).

Some TCI advantages are found. Including cost-effective, secure, quick delivery, easy storage (can be stored!) and easy self-administration.

American researchers tested TCI with Clostridium difficile toxoid A in mice in 2007, with positive results. The bacteria C. Difficult is the leading cause of nosocomial diarrhea, e.g. hospital-infectious diarrhea.

Johns Hopkins University researchers tested TCI's defensive efficacy with enterotoxigenic Escherichia coli (ETEC) heat-labile toxin (LT). Results showed the patch "mediated anti-toxin immune responses that did not prevent but mitigated the disease.

Apollo Life Sciences developed and patented needle-free drug delivery and published preliminary studies on needle-free transdermal delivery of tetanus toxoid vaccine in mice in May 2007.

Apollo has developed TransD, a non-invasive transdermal carrier that works by spreading "a protein-laden water layer across the skin and into the surrounding dermal and subdermal layers.

 It has the potential to replace bio drug injections based on molecules such as interferon, growth hormones and anti-TNF (tumor necrosis factor). "Recently, the TCI produced by biotech firm Iommi, now owned by Austrian company Intercell, made headlines.

Drug Delivery Report explained how it works:" Administration is a two-step process. Next, putting the machine on the patient's arm and removing a tab protects the body.

The tab spreads a slightly abrasive paste across the body, rendering it painless and almost imperceptible, leaving an ink mark to signify where the patch should be applied. The patient then wears an adhesive patch[with the vaccine] for several hours.

"The innovative design firm Ideo helped design the patch which involved removal of an extremely thin skin layer (about one-thousandth of an inch!).

 Currently, Intercell's vaccine patch against traveler diarrhea or so-called Montezuma's Revenge is promising. People could buy this and put it on themselves while they fly. It's the most convenient form of immunization I've ever seen. "

The vaccine was tested on tourists traveling to Guatemala and Mexico and showed 70% effectiveness against traveler diarrhea. In another field study of 170 travelers as part of Phase II vaccine patch trials.

The vaccine patch reduced the risk of moderate to severe traveler diarrhea by 75%. Results of Phase I / II studies showed that a small amount of the vaccine activated a protective immune response in 73% of study participants. Phase II trials were planned in 2009.

Over recent years, vaccine and immunization technology has changed a lot as it tries to meet the health challenges facing developed and developing countries. The TCI or vaccine patch is a groundbreaking device, potentially helping to solve some of the problems facing conventional vaccine delivery systems.

Chapter 9

Vaccines-A Parent's Guide

Children Vaccines lead to a significant reduction in childhood diseases such as Diptheria, Tetanus, Whooping Cough, Polio, Haemophilus Influenzae type-b and, to name a few, Hepatitis B. Families should take the time to learn about vaccine benefits and risks.

Read the possible consequences of not vaccinating against certain diseases. As a service provider, plain language should be used to convey vaccine data and use it to a patient. Printed documentation should also be accessible for any oral explanations.

Parents should know that the risk of a vaccine reaction is much smaller than the risk of serious illness with infectious diseases. Many parents were surprised to learn that children can die of measles, chickenpox, whooping cough and other diseases preventable by vaccines.

 The bacteria and viruses that cause vaccine-preventable diseases and death still exist and can be passed on to non-vaccine-protected people.

Throughout Australia and the United States of America, vaccine coverage is high due to effective vaccination programs. Deaths caused by infant diseases have almost vanished.

Vaccination protects not only individuals but others in the population by increasing the general level of immunity and reducing disease spread. Vaccines may contain life, (attenuated) or killed disease-causing bacteria or viruses.

They cause an immune system response when injected or given by mouth. Vaccines activate the body to make antibodies— proteins that specifically identify and fight the disease that causes bacteria and viruses, and help remove them from the body.

It is important to raise awareness of the proven efficacy of immunization to save lives and prevent serious illness.

Occupational health and safety set strict vaccine development guidelines. Vaccines have the highest safety standards. Each service provider should always have a ready anaphylaxis response package.

Vaccine processing is strictly monitored in refrigerators with a 24-hour temperature monitoring gage. Vaccines transferred from main storage to local hospitals, use the cold-chain transport system.

Diptheria-Can invades the throat, causing dense covering that may cause breathing problems, paralysis, or heart failure.

Tetanus (Lockjaw)—Caused by Clostridium tetani. The bacteria travel from the soil to open wounds and enter the bloodstream. Toxins can cause muscle spasms, lockjaw, speech/breathing trouble, stiffness, and shoulders, back and neck pain.

Whooping Cough-Is caused by highly infectious bacteria spreading by droplets, causing upper respiratory and lung infections. It requires vomiting and' whooping.' Disease symptoms include a lack of brain oxygen contributing to brain damage and possible death.

Polio-Is caused by a virus, and infection signs include headache, nausea and vomiting, weakness, stiffness of neck and back, and severe muscle pain. Polio causes meningitis and paralysis.

Haemophilus Influenzae type b (Hib) — Usually found in the upper respiratory tract (lungs and windpipe), Hib can cause infection in children under 2 years of age because they don't have the antibodies needed to fight this infection.

Hib infection may cause meningitis (a brain and spinal cord infection), epiglottitis (severe throat swelling), arthritis, and pneumonia.

Hepatitis B-Hepatitis B can cause liver infections and damage, hepatitis cancer, and death. Symptoms include exhaustion, fatigue, poor appetite, nausea and vomiting, abdominal discomfort, inflammation, muscle and joint pain, rash, jaundice.

Pneumococcal infections— Streptococcus pneumonia can cause meningitis (membrane infection around the brain and spinal cord), pneumonia, septicemia (blood infection), and middle ear and sinus infections.

Symptoms may include nausea, light sensitivity, stiff neck, weak appetite, fatigue, irritability, and drowsiness. May include fever, vomiting, breathing difficulties.

Varicella (Chickenpox)-Chickenpox is a highly contagious infection caused by the varicella-zoster virus, a member of the herpes virus family. Symptoms can include an open itchy rash, lesions that will crust over.

Complications may include lesion skin infection, scarring, pneumonia, difficulty walking and balancing, meningitis (brain and cord infection), encephalitis (brain infection).

Measles-A highly infectious disease caused by Morbillivirus. This travels from person to person by water droplets. Measles is an illness causing skin rash and flu-like symptoms. Fever, cough, runny nose, and eye inflammation are common symptoms.

Measles complications include eye, brain and lung infections that can cause brain damage and death.

Mumps is a salivary gland disease caused by a virus. Mumps virus spreads by water droplets and infected person's saliva. Common symptoms include fever, headache, swollen glands, especially salivary glands.

It can affect other glands like testicles. Ovaries, pancreas, liver, heart. It can also induce sterility in some men, and some people become deaf.

Rubella (German Measles)-Virus-caused. This virus spreads from person to person by air droplets.

It's skin and lymph node disease. Symptoms may include rash, lymphadenopathy, or joint pain that sometimes leads to arthritis. Rubella infection during pregnancy can cause birth defects.

Meningococcal infections-Caused by several different strains of Neisseria meningitides, it is a serious disease. It is a leading cause of bacterial meningitis in U.S. children aged 2-18. Meningitis is an inflammation of the brain and spinal cord blood.

Septicaemia, pneumonia, inflammation, and conjunctivitis may also occur. Symptoms include high fever, fatigue, nausea, nausea, vomiting, light sensitivity, confusion, irritability, and drowsiness.

Rotavirus-Rotavirus is the most common cause of serious gastroenteritis in infants and young children, causing about half of all gastroenteritis in children under 5 years of age. This viral stomach and intestine infection could cause severe diarrhea and nausea, and fever, leading to severe dehydration.

The disease may start suddenly and in the first few days of the disease, up to one-third of infected children have temperatures above 390 C.

Infection with human papillomavirus (HPV) — Human papillomavirus (HPV) is the name for a group of viruses that cause skin warts, genital warts, and cancer. Many different types of HPV can affect body parts.

 During all types of sexual activity, HPV types that can cause genital warts or cervical cancer can spread by direct skin-to-skin contact with a person with the virus. Cervical cancer signs include irregular and precancerous vaginal and vulvar lesions and genital warts in females aged 9-26. Gardasil's cervical cancer prevention permit.

All of the above are preventable childhood diseases. Common side effects from vaccines include injection site soreness, redness, heat, and swelling, nausea, irritability, drowsiness, mild rash, loss of appetite, muscle aches, diarrhea, and vomiting.

You should notify your health care provider if: your baby has a proven or weakened immune system, is allergic to any of the vaccine's ingredients, or has ever had an allergic reaction after receiving a vaccine dose.

Or if your baby is mildly and severely ill or has responded to neomycin, streptomycin, polymyxin B, gelatin, and eggs.

Vaccination recommended for regular childhood immunization is specified in the National Immunization Program (NIP) schedule and sponsored under the Australia and USA Immunization Program.

Vaccination is a vital step in getting children off to a healthy start and has helped significantly reduce most childhood diseases. Children or adults may be re-vaccinated (with some, but not all, vaccinations) if their immunity from the vaccines drops to a low level or if previous research has shown that long-term safety includes booster vaccination.

It is important to remember that vaccinations are many times healthier than illnesses that avoid Chapter 10 Measles Within the U.S. and Vaccine Avoidance Within the past 5 years, the rise of numerous anti-vaccination campaigns has generated public discussion and vaccination issue concern.

 In a new national CDC study, the percentage of kindergarteners with all available vaccinations varied by the state with coverage as small as 84% in some states to cover more than 99% in other states (with 26 states stating that they did not meet the federally mandated goals of 95% coverage).

Recent widespread measles outbreaks have brought vaccination resistance to the national discussion.

Measles in the U.S. — A Brief History The measles vaccine program began nationally in 1963. Approximately 3 million people contracted measles annually before the program began.

About 400 of that number died, about 48,000 were hospitalized, and over 4,000 developed measles disease encephalitis. In 2000, the CDC declared measles eliminated in the United States. In 2014, the US reported 23 different measles outbreaks Just over 600 cases (383 of these occurred in unvaccinated Ohio communities).

Worldwide, measles is still extremely common and often devastates unvaccinated populations. An estimated 20 million people contract measles each year and 146,000 people die from infection annually (about 17 people an hour).

As of February 6, 2015, the CDC confirms that the U.S. is currently experiencing a large multi-state epidemic that has resulted in 120 outbreaks and is suspected to be related to a California amusement park.

Nevertheless, the virus is similar to the type of virus that caused a large global measles outbreak in the Philippines in 2014.

Measles Transmission: Measles is one of the world's most contagious diseases. Lives in contaminated people's throat and nose mucus and can spread by coughing and sneezing.

Measles may remain in-ground or atmosphere where an infected person sneezed or coughed for up to two hours. It is predicted that 90% of people in close contact with an infected person will develop measles unless otherwise resistant to the disease.

Measles Vaccinations: most people in the developed world are vaccinated (Measles-Mumps-Rubella "MMR vaccine" or "MMRV vaccine").

One dose of a measles vaccine is estimated to be 93% effective in preventing measles (this number rises to 97% after two doses). Accordingly, 3% of all vaccinated individuals can not prevent infection (although infection among these individuals is substantially milder).

A Note on Vaccine Safety: The majority of needed childhood vaccines no longer contain thimerosal or mercury. Policymakers, vaccine manufacturers, and public health officials have called for the elimination or reduction of mercury use within vaccines since the early 2000s.

There are influenza vaccine, Japanese encephalitis, tetanus toxoid, and meningococcal.

Several people have made public statements about the connection between vaccines (specifically measles) and autism.

This hypothesis came from a 1998 study published by a British physician investigating a possible link between autism and measles virus. Subsequent clinical trials could not replicate the original study results and could not create a link between autism and the measles virus.

After a surge of outrage, the paper ultimately dismissed the results, 10 of the 13 original authors removed their names from the report, losing the physician's medical license and being tried for professional misconduct. Recent studies show no correlation between measles and autism.

The largest of these findings were published in the New England Medicine Review, involving a study of over 500,000 children, resulting in no correlation between measles vaccination and autism onset.

Conclusion

Although all current evidence and clinical data show the efficacy of national public vaccination programs, the now statistically significant groups that oppose this view will help bring about a national vaccination debate.

This issue is likely to cause considerable tension between vaccinated children's parents, non-vaccinated children's parents, and public areas where their children may be forced to interact.

To health care providers, the growing threat of malaria cases may bring new challenges to the safe management of at-risk hospital populations.

Here we gave you the top five explanations why you should vaccinate your baby because not having your child vaccinated is like being his biggest enemy.

1. Vaccines keep you safe from illnesses that are not entirely resolved-there are still many diseases and viruses that can cause sickness and death, and can be passed to those who are not covered by vaccines.

During our day, when flying around the globe is just a matter of a few hours, it's not so difficult to see how quickly these viruses could spread around the world.

2. Vaccines keep you safe and protected-Disease and Control Center recommended that people be vaccinated for life-long protection from birth from diseases such as influenza, human papillomavirus, polio, hepatitis A and B.

 But still, most people are not vaccinated, which eventually makes them exposed to these diseases, which can cause chronic illness and sometimes death.

3. Besides exercise and diet, vaccination is also vital-eating, exercising and having a routine medical check-up performed just to test for health conditions such as breast cancer or colon problem, vaccinations do play a very important role in one's health. Vaccines are vital for our health, as they shield us from numerous life-threatening diseases.

4. Vaccination makes a huge difference over the past few years, scientific studies have shown that in 50,000 people die each year in the US due to vaccine-preventable diseases. Vaccinations can make a huge difference in life and death, so it's really important to protect and vaccinate your child.

5. Vaccines are helpful to your body— vaccines are designed to avoid the infection they are made to treat.

Most people have this misconception in mind that vaccinations are the cause of catching disease; well, it's completely untrue, vaccines contain either the "dead" virus or a much-weakened version of the virus so you can't catch and stay safe from it.

Guess you have been enlightened by my Ebook, let me refer you to another of my publications : Casey Anthony: Mother of Disappeared Caylee Anthony"

https://www.amazon.com/Casey-Anthony-Mother-Disappeared-Caylee-ebook/dp/B07QPKJMDN/ref=sr_1_15?keywords=Casey+Anthony&qid=1569776304&s=digital-text&sr=1-15

References

Centers for Disease Control and Prevention. Autism Spectrum Disorder: Data & Statistics. Accessed 01/25/2018.

Rice, C.E., Rosanoff, M., Dawson, G., Durkin, M., Croen, L.A., Singer, A., Yeargin-Allsopp, M. Evaluating changes in the prevalence of the autism spectrum disorders (ASDs).Public Health Reviews. 2012; 34(2): 1.

Hertz-Picciotto, I., Delwiche, L. The rise in autism and the role of age at diagnosis. Epidemiology. 2009; 20(1): 84.

CDC. Autism spectrum disorder (ASD). Research. Accessed 01/25/2018.

National Institutes of Health. National Institute of Neurological Disorders and Stroke. Autism spectrum disorder fact sheet. Accessed 01/25/2018.

Immunization Safety Review Committee, Institute of Medicine. Immunization safety review: vaccines and autism. National Academies Press, 2004. Accessed 01/25/2018.

Thompson, N.P., Pounder, R.E., Wakefield, A.J., & Montgomery, S.M. Is measles vaccination a risk factor for inflammatory bowel disease? The Lancet. 1995; 345(8957): 1071-1074.

Fudenberg, H.H. Dialysable lymphocyte extract (DLyE) in infantile onset autism: a pilot study. Biotherapy. 1996; 9(1-3): 143-147.

Gupta, S. Immunology and immunologic treatment of autism. Proc Natl Autism Assn Chicago.1996;455–460

Wakefield A, et al. RETRACTED:—Ileal-lymphoid-nodular hyperplasia, non-specific colitis, and pervasive developmental disorder in children. Lancet. 1998; 351(9103): 637-641.

Deer, B. Royal free facilitates attack on MMR in medical school single shots videotape. No date. Accessed 01/25/2018.

Deer, B. Revealed: Wakefield's secret first MMR patent claims "safer measles vaccine." No date. Accessed 01/25/2018.

Offit, P.A. Autism's False Profits. New York: Columbia University Press; 2008. See Chapters 2 and 3.

See a list of such studies in this Children's Hospital of Philadelphia Vaccine Education Center document.

Horton, R. A statement by the editors of The Lancet. The Lancet. 2004; 363(9411): 820-821.

Laurance, J. How was the MMR scare sustained for so long when the evidence showed that it was unfounded? The Independent. September 19, 2004. Accessed 01/25/2018.

Murch, S.H., Anthony, A., Casson, D.H., Malik, M., Berelowitz, M., Dhillon, A.P., … Walker-Smith, J.A. Retraction of an interpretation. Lancet. 2004; 363(9411): 750.

The Editors of The Lancet. Comment: RETRACTION:—Ileal-lymphoid-nodular hyperplasia, non-specific colitis, and pervasive developmental disorder in children. The Lancet. 2010; 375(9713): 445. Accessed 01/25/2018.

Meikle, J., Boseley, S. MMR row doctor Andrew Wakefield struck off register. May 24, 2010. Accessed 01/25/2018.

Deer, B. How the case against the MMR vaccine was fixed. BMJ. 2011; 342: c5347. Accessed 01/25/2018.

Godlee, F., Smith, J., Marcovitch, H. Wakefield's article linking MMR vaccine and autism was fraudulent. BMJ. 2011; 342: c7452. Accessed 01/25/2018.

World Health Organization. Thimerosal in vaccines. July 2006. Accessed 01/25/2018.

Most of this narrative refers to the facts and chronology outlined in the Food and Drug Administration's Publication Thimerosal in Vaccines.

Immunization Safety Review Committee, Institute of Medicine. (2001). Immunization safety review: measles-mumps-rubella vaccine and autism. National Academies Press. Accessed 01/25/2018.

CDC. Science summary: CDC studies on vaccines and autism. Accessed 01/25/2018.

American Academy of Pediatrics. Vaccine safety: examine the evidence. (122KB). Updated April 2013. Accessed 01/25/2018.

DeStefano, F., Price, C.S., Weintraub, E.S. Increasing exposure to antibody-stimulating proteins and polysaccharides in vaccines is not associated with risk of autism. The Journal of Pediatrics. 2013; 163(2): 561-567.

Children's Hospital of Philadelphia. Vaccine Education Center. Vaccines ingredients: Aluminum. Accessed 01/25/2018.

CDC. Autism spectrum disorder (ASD). Research. Accessed 01/25/2018.

National Institutes of Health. National Institute of Neurological Disorders and Stroke. Autism spectrum disorder fact sheet. Accessed 01/25/2018.